5 Inches

The diary of a very small penis

By Ivan Small

Published by Robin Barratt
© Ivan Small 2015

ISBN: 978-1514773833

W: www.RobinBarrattPublishing.com
E: Robin@RobinBarrattPublishing.com
E: RobinBarratt@yahoo.com

"My boyfriend has a tiny poke,
otherwise he's a real good bloke"
Anonymous

Alabama black snake, anaconda, anal impaler, baby arm, baby maker, bald-headed yogurt slinger, baloney, pony, BBC, BBD, big Dick and the twins, big Italian salami, bird, bobby, dangler, bologna, pony, bone, boner, boom stick, bratwurst, broner, bud, cack, chap, choad, chode, chopper, chub, chubbie, chup, chut, cock, cock rocket, cornholer, cut, D, dangler, dick, dick smalls, ding, ding-a-ling, ding dong, dingis, dinker, dinky, dipstick, disco stick, doder, doinker, domepiece, dong, dork, general, two colonels, get it up, giggle stick, gut wrench, hard-on, head, helmet, hockey cocky, hog, hooded, hotdog, hung, jimmy, johnson, John Thomas, joystick, kielbasa, knob, lady boner, love muscle, love shaft, love stick, main vein, manhood, man muscle, master of ceremonies, meat popsicle, meat thermometer, member, middle leg monster, Mr. Happy, Mr. Winky, ol' one-eye, one-eyed monster, one-eyed snake, one-eyed trouser snake, P, packer, patz, pecker, peen, pee pee, peeper, peeter, Peter, Ph.D, pickle, piece, pink tractor beam, plonker, pocket rocket, polaroid, pole, pop a chub, pork sword, prick, pud, purple-headed soldier, purple headed solider man, purple-headed warrior, putz, rod, Russell the love muscle, salami, sausage, schlong, schlort, schmeckel, schwartz, sconge, shaft, shlittle, shlong, shrinkage, skin flute, steamin' semen roadway, stiffie, stiffy, tallywacker, tallywhacker, tally whacker, tent pole, thing, third leg, throbber, tonsil tickler, tool, tripod, trouser meat, trouser snake, tube steak, twig, unit, wang, wanker, wankie, wee, weenie, wee wee, weiner, whang, whiskey dick, who who dilly, wiener, willie, willy, winky, wood, yogurt slinger, yoo-hoo, zubra.

INTRODUCTION

My small penis has, over most of my adult lifetime, caused me considerably stress and deep emotional anxiety. It has affected how I feel about myself, my sex life and how I interact with other people. It is tough, really tough having a smaller than average cock; no one takes the piss out of small boobs or a small bum, but everyone, everyone, takes the piss out of a small penis and even mentioning having a small cock, or writing about having a small cock causes most people to grin and snigger. My physicality has also caused me to seriously consider taking my own life, yet people still find it funny.

And so I thought I'd tell my story about what I have gone through (and still do), over the years and how having a smaller than average manhood has affected me. There are no penis anxiety solutions in this book though, it is just my own personal story about what I have been through and what I think and feel, in the hope of firstly sharing my story with other people around the world with the same physicality in order to show them that they are not alone, and secondly to perhaps try to make people understand the deep emotional scares that having a small penis can cause, and how taking the piss out of someone smaller than average can, and often does, have lasting and quite possibly devastating consequences.

Although this book is quite sad in places, I have tried to be humorous too, as well as add a few interesting (well, I found them interesting) facts about the penis and penis worship.

Honestly, I am not sure if I will ever accept myself as I am, and I think I will go to my grave always being acutely embarrassed about what I have (or rather have not), down below, as well as despising what I have and wishing so much I was different. I know that I might also go to my grave never being physically adored either. There is no physical solution to my problem, and emotionally I think I am just too scarred to change.

Best wishes

Ivan
Please feel free to contact me via my publisher:
IvanSmall@RobinBarrattPublishing.com

CONTENTS

SIZE MATTERS... REALLY, IT DOES!

They say size doesn't matter, but that's nonsense. Believe me, it matters! Most women would agree that a cock slightly under five inches (12.7 centimetres) erect is probably a little too small and, as one women very honestly and openly said to me once; *"Women don't fantasize about small cocks!"* It's true, they don't. They don't close their eyes and imagine a tiny little cock slightly less than five inches erect bouncing towards them, they imagine a big, thick cock. They don't imagine a small cock in their hand or mouth or in their pussy, they imagine a large one.

A big cock is undeniably aesthetically stunning and commanding; it is something to behold, to stare at and to admire. A big cock fascinates almost everyone; men and women, young and old, and the allure and attraction of size is a symbol of arousal, and anyone saying any different is either lying to you, or not wanting to hurt you... if you're small. People love looking at big cocks, and if a woman had the choice of a seven inch (17.78 centimetres) cock inside her, or a cock less than five inches, she would take the seven inch cock any day. Most women like the feeling of being filled and larger cocks fill, small ones don't. Physically size matters.

Of course you can be a great lover with a tiny cock, and a terrible lover with a big cock, as women everywhere constantly try to assure us, as they also try to assure us, time and time again, that size really doesn't matter. But what about being a great lover with a big cock? This is what fantasies are made of; great lovers with great big cocks. Porn is fantasy, fantasy mainly made by men, for men, featuring big cocks, not small ones. There are no best-selling porn films featuring men with small cocks! Erotica is much milder and a lot more subtle sexual fantasy, which women mostly tend write, read and watch, and again features men who are hung. I've read a little erotica, as I prefer the subtleness of it compared to in-your-face porn, but I have never read any stories where a man takes out his tiny cock, or she looks down at his beautiful yet tiny cock, or she guides his tiny cock inside her. Aside from humorous erotica, where men with small cocks make people laugh, or denigrating erotica where men with small cocks are something to be laughed at. Women don't read erotica and close their eyes and fantasize about men with cocks, they are not interested and it doesn't arouse them. They are interested in reading about, and fantasizing about, and being aroused by men who are well-endowed.

When writing this little book, I put an anonymous question on an online sex forum about size, asking people to be completely honest and open about what is too big for a cock, and what is too small. I only left it online for about forty-eight hours and in that time a little over one hundred women replied! Almost everyone said that, physically, size does indeed matter, even if they have pretended to themselves, and to others, that it didn't. I am not talking about love, but purely from a physical basis, almost every woman said that a bigger than average cock is much better and more arousing than a smaller than average cock. Another recent survey said exactly the same thing; that women did indeed prefer big penises, but not too big. And a three inch (7.6 cm) flaccid penis was the size most women preferred to look at when showed pictures of naked men. Studies also show that women who orgasm through vaginal stimulation were much more fussy about penis size than other women; larger cocks make them orgasm eighty percent more frequently than with a small one. Physiologically, size matters too as, according to researchers at the State University of New York, the longer your penis, the better semen displacement you'll achieve when having sex with a woman flush with competing sperm. If that's what you do on a regular basis! They used artificial phalluses to test the scooping mechanism of the penis's coronal ridge, which is apparently designed to get rid of other men's semen so that your semen has a better chance of fertilizing the woman. Now that's one hell of a research programme.

Women together talk about cock size. It's a fact, and even the most respectable women in all walks of life and occupations, gossip about cocks and cock size; *"Did he have a big cock?"*, *"No, he was tiny!"* laughter all around. Or; *"Yes, he was huge!"* followed by shrieks of excitement, blushes and giggles, and hands and palms measuring the approximate size of it, followed by more laughter and soft sighs of envy. Women seem very happy to mention to their friends if their man is well-endowed, but they most definitely keep it to themselves if he isn't, especially if he's tiny. A boyfriend with a tiny cock? That's something never to mention... to anyone. I saw a Facebook post recently from a women posting a picture of her boyfriend in the gym wearing tight Lycra shorts, accentuating his undeniably big cock. She was jokingly boasting about his size and thickness and her picture of him and his cock had loads and loads (and loads!) of 'lucky girl' comments. She had no hesitation at all about sharing her boyfriend's cock size with all her friends on Facebook - and I'm anyone else that was interested. I bet she wouldn't do that if he was tiny; she wouldn't tell anyone!

I saw another picture on Facebook of an obviously well-endowed man in his briefs, and was astonished at the hundreds, yes hundreds, of 'wow, lucky him' comments from women - and surprisingly a few men - below the picture. Some comments disturbingly obscene. Men who are hung are considered lucky, attractive, desired and sexy and, from the comments of many of the girls, most definitely wanted; most women commenting seem to want a man hung like that. Men with small cocks? Quite the opposite; not particularly desired, attractive or sexy. I don't think that there would be the same sorts of comments, or even the same amount of comments if there was a picture of someone with an obviously tiny cock. Actually, I can imagine there would be quite a few very nasty, unkind and cruel comments.

And if a man who is hung is lucky, does this mean that a man who isn't hung is unlucky? Does he somehow become unattractive? Not particularly desired or wanted? Does he become something to be laughed at and to be ridiculed? In this modern Western society, of course he does! In this society, a man isn't a real man if he hasn't got a big cock. But not so for the man who isn't hung. A real man has a big cock, after all, cock are called '*man*hood' and for a reason. It has also been proven in many sexual surveys that men with bigger than average cocks are also more promiscuous; a man who is hung knows what he's got, he's proud with what he's got in his pants and he's not shy either in showing it off. Men with small cocks have far fewer sexual partners. No man wants a small cock, and no one wants a man with a small cock.

And of course there are the cock innuendos and size-matters puns and jokes that abound just about everywhere; in newspapers and magazines, in films and television programmes and on talk-shows, and a few months ago I even went to a friend's child's school pantomime of *Robin Hood* where I counted at least three 'size-counts' innuendos... yes even at a pantomime with kids as young as seven and eight there are implications that the size of a man's manhood is important. And how many women have you seen giving the little-finger sign when describing a person with a tiny cock? And we have all heard the 'big car, small cock' phrase, and just about everyone's email in-boxes are full of 'get a bigger and thicker cock' spam messages. Cocks and cock size is everywhere.

And women wonder why men are so centred on the size of their cock, when society itself is so focused on cocks and cock-size! Women are just as focused on body-shape and boobs and bum as men are about the size of their cock, and for exactly the same reasons; women's bodies and having the perfect body-shape are sexualised everywhere, and so is having the perfect cock.

Of course, it's true that women don't wait around for that one perfect man with that one perfect penis, and most sex surveys show that actually around eight-five percent of women are satisfied with the penis size of their partners (although only fifty percent of men are happy with their own size) but, as another women once said to me; *"Cock size isn't that important, but having a man with a big cock is certainly a bonus!"*

MY COCK IS A LITTLE UNDER FIVE INCHES LONG

My cock is a little under five inches long when erect; four and three-quarter inches (12.06 centimetres) to be exact. I have measured it... many times! Soft it is just over an inch, and it's just over five inches around the girth too.

There are two types of penises; the first is a penis that is small when flaccid but expands and lengthens when becoming erect. This is called a *Grower*. The second type of penis appears big when flaccid, but doesn't get much bigger when erect. This is called a *Shower* (as in 'to show' and not to shower!). I am a grower as, at just over an inch, mine looks tiny when flaccid and grows over four times bigger when erect.

If you want to know what four and three-quarter inches are like, take out your smart phone; they are usually a little under five inches, roughly the same as my penis erect. Or slightly shorter than the width of a standard paperback book. Or, even better, take out a tape-measure and measure four and three-quarter inches. It isn't very big. This means I am not normal; only around two percent of Western men have a penis size in this category.

I hate the size of my cock. I am often embarrassed by it and have occasionally been ridiculed because of it. I have even thought about taking my life because of it; because that would be the one and only true way of never again going through the trauma and stress of getting emotionally involved with someone, and therefore getting intimate with someone, and therefore possibly getting ridiculed or laughed at, again.

Sad isn't it?

There are many, many cock-size surveys, both under strict medical conditions for sexual health research, as well as more general, global surveys by websites and commercial organisations such as the condom makers Durex.

One of the first such studies was in 1948, when the Kinsey Institute conducted a pioneering study on erect penis size for a book titled: *Sexual Behaviour in Human Male.* One of the first ever surveys on sexuality, they measured the size of three thousand, five hundred erections, and the results from this very first survey on penis length showed that the average (65.7%) range of penis size when erect was between 5.5 and 6.5 inches, with the mean length slightly over six inches (15.24 centimetres). It also showed that only one man out of a hundred measured eight inches (20.32 centimetres), only seven men in a thousand had erections larger than eight inches, and only one man out of a thousand had an erect penis larger than nine inches (22.86 centimetres). They didn't measure each and every individual cocks themselves though; they gave the person being measured a card, with measurements along its side, which was then to be placed against the erect cock and a mark was made at the appropriate place. The statistics were not perhaps as reliable as they could have been, as people might have been inclined to exaggerate a little when measuring themselves, or indeed not measuring themselves properly. A short while later though, Kinsey wanted to update the research and actually measured the erections of three hundred volunteers, which gave a slightly different average length of between 5.5 inches and six inches.

In a more recent Durex survey, the average erection globally was shown to be 6.4 inches, but this survey showed that there were in fact quite a few more men with much larger cocks than in the earlier Kinsey report; four to seven men per hundred with eight inch erections, thirty to forty men per thousand with erections of nine inches, and between ten and thirty men per thousand with erections larger than nine inches.

Another survey was recently conducted and published in the British newspaper *The Guardian* which measured the penises of fifteen thousand men. That's a lot of penises! I am not sure how all these cocks were measured, as I can't imagine anyone actually physical measuring fifteen thousand cocks. What a job that would be! This particular survey showed the average length when erect was a lot smaller, at just 5.16 inches (13.12 centimetres). After releasing these statistics the report summarised; *"The numbers should help reassure the large majority of men that the size of their penis is in the normal range, and can be used to help men with small penis anxiety."* At 4.75 inches, my erection is still much smaller than the average of 5.16 inches! This survey also found that only 2.28% of the male population has an unusually small penis of under five inches, and the same percentage of men had an unusually large erection of over eight inches.

However, another size survey conducted by The-Penis.com found the average erect length to be 5.9 inches, with slight variations in region; for example African and Arab men's cocks are on average one, to one and a half inches bigger - between 6.5 and 7.5 inches erect, with an average Arab man's cock measuring between 7.2 and 7.6 inches. Indian and Asian men's cocks were on average slightly smaller, between five and 5.5 inches erect. This was confirmed in another global survey which showed the smallest cocks in the world belonged to North Korean men, at an average erect length of 3.8 inches (9.65 centimetres). In South Korea however, the average penis length is slightly longer, at 4.3 inches (10.92 centimetres) [could this be the *real* reason why North Korean's mad, megalomaniac leader Kim Jong-un is still officially at war with South Korea? Because South Koreans have bigger cocks then he does? Actually, not just South Korea, but most of the rest of the world has a bigger cock that he does! Penis envy at the extreme]. The next smallest erections are with men from India and Thailand with an average erect cock length of four inches (10.16 centimetres). The biggest average cocks in the world are to be found in the Democratic Republic of the Congo, where the average erection length is 7.1 inches, then Equator at 6.9 inches, and Columbia and Venezuela at 6.7 inches. This survey shows the largest average

European size are Italian and French cocks who measure in at an average 6.2 inches erect, with British cocks averaging 5.5 inches.

So, after all these different surveys, I think we can safely come to the conclusion that, in the West anyway, the average cock size when erect is about six inches, give or take a quarter or so of an inch. And in general though, just a very small percentage of the population are over eight inches erect and, as mentioned, and a little over two percent of the population surveyed are under five inches erect.

You may ask what's an extra inch and a half? But actually, to a man with a smaller than average cock, it's a lot! If you took a tape measure and put it against your groin and then measure out four and three quarter inches, and then six inches, there is indeed quite a difference. Then, for a laugh, measure out 13.5 inches (34.29 centimetres) for John Falcon's cock.

BIG COCKS AND SMALL PUSSIES

But why is society so focused on the size of men's cocks? And why are men with small cocks so continually ridiculed, humiliated and laughed at? These are rhetorical questions, because honestly I really don't know. It's sad though, and it really doesn't make any sense because men never talk about big or small pussies; you never hear 'size counts' (or doesn't) when it comes to a woman's pussy. You never hear a group of men talking about pussy size: "Did she have a big pussy?" , "No, she was tiny!" laughter all around. And of course the media never mentions pussy size as they do so often with cock size, and you never see men imitating the size of a woman's vagina as women do with the size of a man's penis, in fact this would be considered by just about everyone as pretty repulsive. And if a man did talk about the size of a woman's pussy as openly as women talk about the size of a man's cock, he would undoubtedly be called just about ever obscenity under-the-sun, and might even be arrested (I am sure the would be a crime under the obscenity law for such a thing). A man openly talking about the size of a woman's pussy would be considered by most as both disgusting and offensive. And consider the consequences and repercussions if the media and films, and television talk-show hosts joked as openly about pussy size as they do about cock size? Programmes would be banned, programme makers and hosts probably sacked - and quite possibly arrested - and I am sure production company offices would even be picketed by enraged women. So why is talking and joking about cocks and the sizes of cocks so funny and revered and acceptable, and yet talking and joking about pussy size sick, obscene and objectionable? And yet women, and society, do talk openly and freely about cocks with relative impunity.

I saw an ITV *This Morning* programme talking to a man who already had a ten inch (25.4 centimetres) cock, but then went onto have an operation to make it even bigger. When asked if size counts, he said there were some women who thought he was just too big for them, but most women loved his cock. "Women," he said, "love big cocks."

I also once saw an trailer for another ITV *This Morning* programme interviewing John Falcon. I didn't actually watch the programme, but at 13.5 inches (34.29 centimetres) erect, John is a celebrity in his home city of New York because he has the world's largest penis. Yes, he's a celebrity just because of the size of his cock! His cock is three times longer than my cock but somehow can't see me becoming a celebrity because of the small size my cock! The *Daily Mail* then wrote about this show: *"Measuring eight inches when flaccid and an impressive 13.5 inches when erect, the 41 year-old's XL asset hit the headlines recently when the huge bulge in his trousers caused a security alert at San Francisco airport."* And yet I don't think there would ever be a programme about the biggest ever recorded vagina in the world, and would the *Daily Mail* write about a huge woman's vagina as being impressive? Certainly not! Nor I doubt, in this politically correct world, would they even write about woman's boobs as being impressive either. So why is it okay to still write about a cock as being impressive?

Saying that though, I also saw that there was an ITV *This Morning* programme (what's this about *The Morning* and cocks?) interviewing Patrick Moote, whose video went viral of his girlfriend turning down his marriage proposal at a basketball game because he had a small penis. He said to the show's co-hosts Phillip Schofield and Amanda Holden; *"She told me I was a little too small for her."*

However, I did see on Oddee.com that the world's biggest vagina most likely belonged to Scottish giantess Anna Swan (1846-1888), who apparently set a number of records relating to her size. Born normal sized, she began growing at a exceptional rate in childhood, finally reaching a maximum height of 7' 8" (2.33 metres) at age nineteen. But, if she lived today, I don't think she'd be interviewed anywhere about her very large vagina!

IS HAVING A SMALL COCK A PHYSICAL DISABILITY?

Of course, you can love a person whatever their physicality, and I don't think there are many people in the world that would say any different; people with all sorts of differing physicalities and disabilities that shift away from the 'normal,' find love and adoration and happiness. This is undeniable. And most partners of the disabled would say that they don't care at all about someone's physical differences and disabilities, even if they can sometimes be challenging, because it is the person they love, not what they are like physically. And I won't deny this either; it is the person and what his or her heart and soul is like that is infinitely more important to most sincere people than what they look like, or what physical disabilities and challenges they might have, or the size of their cock. There are the very superficial though that just care about looks and perfection, and who wouldn't dream of having a partner, less than perfect looking, but I like to think that they are in the minority and that most people are not like this.

But what does the person with an 'abnormal' physicality actually think and feel about themselves?

I remember a friend of mine had a testicle removed because of cancer. It almost wrecked his fifteen year marriage. I knew the couple very well, and many times his wife said to me that she didn't care at all about him losing one. Of course she didn't, she would love him despite his physicality. But she failed to see things through his eyes, which almost cost them their marriage; because *he* cared terribly about how *he* looked. At one point things got really bad between them and they were almost on the edge of separating. But once she started to understand how he felt, and saw things through his eyes and understood how he saw himself, things slowly started to change and thankfully, many years later, they are still together.

Another very pretty girl friend of mine is completely flat-chested. Completely. Her devoted boyfriend doesn't care, not in the slightest. Why would he? He loves her dearly whether she had big boobs or no boobs. But *she* cares about how *she* looks, a lot, and whenever they are out and about and dressed up, she would get a little jealous and depressed if she noticed him looking at other women's busts, even if just fleetingly or inadvertently. Some busts you can't help but notice! For her; her bust is a really big deal. She is so pretty and has such a lovely personality, but she hates her body and she hates how she looks, and she constantly compares herself to other women with bigger busts. She sees other women with bigger busts as a threat. She would love to have breast augmentation surgery, but she can't afford it. And anyway, her boyfriend is dead against her having bits of plastic on her chest.

And this is exactly how I feel about my cock.

Like any disability or unusual physicality, it isn't necessarily what others think of you that really matters, as much as what you think of yourself.

Having a very small cock is abnormal, because it isn't normal, and anything not normal is by default abnormal. Is it a disability too because, as with some other disabilities, having a small cock can and does cause some real physical, sexual and emotional challenges.

And if a physical disability causes emotional and physical distress, why is it acceptable for some people to then be so public and open about this disability? Taking the piss out of someone with a facial disfigurement, or in a wheel-chair, or with other physical disabilities is considered disrespectful and offensive, but somehow taking the piss out of someone with a small cock is acceptable. Why is this? Is it because it is sexual and anything sexual can be funny? Is it because it isn't as obvious a disability as perhaps other physical disabilities? Or maybe it is because it isn't recognised as being a disability? Or maybe because it is anonymous, and that 'size' jokes and innuendos are not normally aimed at anyone in particular, but just generally to everyone with a small penis.

Some people reading this little book about cock size might just laugh and say that I should not be so ridiculous and stupid, and to 'get a life' and to accept myself for who I am, even if this physicality does indeed cause real and deep emotional stress, as well as obvious sexual challenges. And maybe there really are many, many women that will simply say that honestly, from their hearts, having a small cock really doesn't matter because it is what you do with it that counts, and not its size. And maybe there are also some women out there who have never, ever taken the piss out of small cocks or someone with a small cock, nor ever would. If you are one of those women, from my heart, thank you! But I also know that there are lots of women who would openly say it doesn't matter that a man has a small one, when in fact they know in their hearts that it does matter; that larger cocks are indeed physically better than smaller ones. And there are also lots of women who may say that they haven't ever taken the piss out of someone with a small cock, or laughed with their friends about someone with a small cock, but in their hearts they know that actually they have. People lie, they then defend those lies as the truth, even though they know it to be a lie. This is human nature.

GETTING IT BIGGER

I have tried many things to increase the length and thickness of my cock, but so far nothing has worked. I used a vacuum pump every day, twice a day, for about three months. Actually, I got through three different vacuum pumps, as the plastic casing in all three started to crack and eventually they all fell apart! Seriously! So either I was pumping too hard, in the vain hope of seeing some massive gains in size, or they were just not up to the task of increasing the size of such a small cock. When I pumped, my cock grew quite significantly inside the chamber, which was great to see; I really loved seeing its new size and thickness inside the vacuum, and it even got to just under six inches as I frantically pumped away (probably why I got through so many appliances), but this increase dissipated a few seconds after using the pump, and it was back to my normal size. They were never any permanent gains, even after using the pump twice daily for three months, my cock remained just about 4.75 inches when erect.

I have tried thickening creams too, no change either. All they did was get me hard and, because of the sensation of the cream over my manhood, make me want to masturbate. Not a bad thing I suppose, but not what I bought it for.

I once even foolishly bought 'get big' tablets advertised in a well-known men's lifestyle magazine, bizarrely thinking that perhaps taking a few tablets every day will do the trick. Three months worth, sixty pounds I think I spent on them! Waste of money, not sure what they did but they had no affect on my penis at all.

I have used a cock ring on occasions too, as I had a short-term relationship with a girl who wanted to try one on me to see if it made me any bigger and thicker. It did increase the girth a little; she said she noticed it was a little thicker, but it didn't affect the length. Nothing I have tried so far has affected my length.

I have also seriously thought about surgery, but I just don't have the money. There are two operations available to increase penis size; the first involves cutting the suspensory ligament which joins the penis to the pelvic area, and supports the penis in an upright position when it's erect. When the ligament is cut, the penis hangs lower, which can therefore make it look longer. However, cutting the ligament may also cause the penis to point more downwards when erect and, although small, I do like it to stand up when erect and not pointing to the floor. It's all very well having a slightly bigger cock, but that's no good if a woman is waiting for it to get erect when it is in fact already erect but just pointing to the floor. Also, a study in 2006 found that this particular procedure led to an average increase of only half an inch in penis length when flaccid, but only a little over a quarter of the men who had the operation were happy with the results. That isn't many people, and obviously means a little under three quarters were not happy. Actually, I can understand why; a half and inch and a downward pointing cock isn't a life-changer! And anyway, a half an inch will take my cock to just over five inches, which is still too small and won't make any difference at all in how I feel about it or about myself. I don't want a half and inch, I want to be at least average with a six inch erect cock. In this regard, I want to be normal and have normal sex and a normal sex life and feel comfortable and confident sexually.

There is another operation called penoplasty, where fat is taken from other parts of the body and put into the cock making it thicker. It is expensive, around 10,000 GBP, and there's a real risk that the penis may look uneven or lumpy, and there may be scarring too. I have enough emotional and physical challenges with the cock I have, let alone a lumpy and scarred one! Also, the injected fat can disappear over time as the body slowly re-absorbs it, so it could be that after feeling great about having that little extra thickness, my cock eventually returns to its previous small size. I'll also be ten grand lighter too!

COME ON BIG BOY, SHOW ME WHAT YOU'RE MADE OF!

I am quite a big built guy; just under six foot (1.82 metres) tall and, at a little under seventeen store (106 kilo), quite muscular. Because of this, women expect a big cock. I am a big man and so I should have a big cock, right? But, whenever I *have* allowed things get intimate with a woman, I can see and sense their disappointment as they see I don't have a big cock at all, in fact I have a tiny one! Of course most women would deny that they feel disappointed, but I, (and they), know the truth. Some women have been lovely though, and have made me feel okay about myself and about my physicality, which is nice, even if, as mentioned earlier, it makes no difference at all as to how I feel about myself. But some women have been just plain nasty and hurtful and horrible about my cock. And it is these hurtful comments that have stayed with me and have scarred and tormented me and that have, over time, destroyed my self-worth and self-confidence. And it is these comments that have made it so very hard for me to get intimate with anyone, for fear of being ridiculed and humiliated.

I have to say that, despite my penis size, I have been lucky because, over my lifetime, I have been adored. Emotionally adored, but never physically. I have always yearned to be physically adored too. I was married for twelve years and, during that time, she would almost never see me naked; I would get changed as quickly as I could, always making sure she and I were in different rooms or when she was in the bathroom, so she wouldn't see my penis, and I would never walk around naked in front of her, ever! I was always so embarrassed about my little one inch cock, just dangling there. Yuck. We were rarely intimate either, she loved me but she didn't love my cock and would rarely touch it or play with it, and she almost never had oral sex with me. It was mainly me performing oral sex on her and then intercourse and little else. During those twelve years she almost never saw me erect.

I use weights and go to the gym almost ever day, but I never use the communal changing rooms or showers either, and never naked around other men changing. And if I did want to use the shower cubicles, I would always make sure I changed into my underwear in the shower cubicle itself, and not in the actual changing area. Not only am I acutely self-concious in front of women for fear of ridicule, I am self-concious in front of everyone! I had to stay in hospital for about a week once, and was even frightened of the nurses seeing my bits, the thought of it terrified me.

As a teenager I didn't really realise I had such a small cock though, mainly because I hadn't seen any other erect cocks to compare mine too, and therefore thought I was fairly normal. There was no Internet when I was growing up, so it was mainly magazine porn, more specifically *Whitehouse* magazine, which bizarrely marketed itself as a sex-education publication. *Whitehouse* first went to press in 1974 and was ironically named after the anti-porn campaigner Mary Whitehouse. It was first available from the top shelves of newsagents, but disappeared from these shelves as it got more and more explicit. It finally disappeared altogether and the company folded as the Internet offered virtually everyone free access to porn. I remember someone bringing a copy of *Whitehouse* into school though, and us teenagers huddled around the magazine flicking through its sordid pages at school break. Personally, as a teenager, I could never get hold of porns as these magazines were, of course, only sold to adults, and I never had a stash under my bed as some other teenagers I knew did, so I suppose the friend who brought it into school stole it from his parents. Bizarrely though, as I studied the pages and these huge cocks in the magazine, I somehow thought that my cock was roughly the same size! True, some men's cocks did seem to look a little bigger than mine, but somehow in my eyes, the majority seemed roughly the same size. I don't know why I thought this, but I did! Plus I don't remember seeing any porn films either up until probably my very late teens or early twenties, so again I didn't have any other much larger cocks to compare mine too. So, from my perspective anyway, and not really knowing any different, I genuinely believed my cock was roughly normal and average and a bit like most other cocks, until I met a girl one night and she looked at my little erection and said; *"Fuck, it's tiny!"* Only then did I really understand that perhaps I was a lot smaller than most.

I remember another time, again when I was roughly the same age. I had met a girl in a bar and taken her home. As soon as we got into the door she quickly stripped off, sat on the bed naked, opened her legs and said; *"Come on big boy, show me what you're made of."* Really, I'm not making it up. She really did open her legs and say this! No stress then! After being called tiny a few months previously, I was nervous, shy and pretty ashamed at my erection, but I got undressed anyway and, standing there naked and erect, she then said; *"Oh, Not made of much then!"* I can't really remember what happened after she said that, because it was such a long time ago and I was probably a tad drunk at the time too, but I do know nothing intimate happened between us.

And another time I was humiliated, although admittedly not really intentionally, was about a year later when a girl dumped her boyfriend to be with me. I can't really remember how we first met, but we were friend's at first and had chatted and had met for coffee a few times and she had already told me she hadn't been happy with him for a long while. One evening we went out – just as friends - for a drink, came back to my bedsit, got kissing and, as things do, one thing led to another. I was so nervous, as the last two times at trying to get my little end away hadn't ended well, but I allowed her hands to touch me and caress me. She fumbled a bit, and then she stopped and said: *"I'm so, so sorry, but I don't really know what to do with it, it's so small."* I think I was probably physically sick after she said that to me, although I do believe she didn't mean to upset me as much as she did, and she was really apologetic.

It was then though that I think I really changed.

After all those those horrible, hurtful words, I didn't want anyone to ever see or touch my tiny cock again. I felt disfigured in some way, not normal, not natural. I wanted so much to be normal, to be sexually desired but my heart sank knowing that I would never be, not physically desired anyway.

GREAT BODY, HANDSOME, BUT WITH A TINY COCK

Without bragging, I was very good looking when I was younger. I knew that, although I was unsure of myself, quite shy and never arrogant with my looks. I was quite ironic really; because I knew that women turned their heads towards me and looked at me when I entered a pub or club, or even just out and about. I was even offered a male modelling job with a well-known London modelling agency. I had no trouble meeting women, and some really beautiful women at that, but I was painfully shy and couldn't understand at all what anyone saw in me. At my age now things are a little different of course, age changes a person's pretty-boy good looks, and not always for the better! but some of the women I met when I was a lot younger were really stunning. However, because of how I felt about myself and my body, I would very rarely go any further than being just friends, and almost never intimate. Not because I didn't want to. Of course I did! And not because I didn't fancy them either, because I did; perfect looks, perfect body, what was there not to fancy? But because I was often so ashamed at my physicality and I didn't want to ever go through the same humiliating experiences that I had previously went through. Quite simply; I was embarrassed with my cock.

I can honestly say I hated my penis, and if ever I did let my guard down and get intimate with someone, I couldn't help thinking that the woman I was with was comparing my tiny cock with the larger cocks of their previous partners. Even if they denied it openly, I know that most women compare the size of their lovers' manhoods! We all compare; maybe not openly or consciously, but we all compare, as we all then use that comparison as points of reference in almost everything we do. Comparison is part of our daily lives. And I know that women compare my cock to other cocks, as mine is significantly smaller than most others!

One woman said to me once; *"Honestly, yes it's small, the smallest I have seen actually, but it's you I really like, not your cock,"* which was, of course, a very nice, kind thing for her to say but demonstrates how women do indeed compare cocks, as, I suppose, men might compare busts and bums. But not pussies. I don't think men compare pussies and men don't humiliate women about their bust, or bum or pussy as some women humiliate men about their cock. As I mentioned, my flat-chested girl friend is adored by her boyfriend but that doesn't change the way she feels about herself.

Even though I am no longer as handsome as I once was when I was much younger (who is?), I do still meet women and I still yearn to get physically close to them and to be intimate. I still want to be loved and adored. Who doesn't? And getting older hasn't stopped these emotions and natural needs and desires. But, when a woman's hands slowly go down towards my cock I usually say; *"Let's go slower,"* or *"I'm not quite ready."* And because of this, women have either thought it was because I didn't fancy them sexually, which of course it wasn't, or that I wanted to know them better before we got intimate, which actually happens to be very true because in my mind, if I think a women really likes me for me, and who I am, and my character and personality, and that I am kind and generous and loving, she might not then be bothered about what I have, or rather haven't, in the trouser department. But even so, as I get to know people and as things get a little more intimate, in the forefront of my mind there is always an absolutely belief she will laugh at me or make some rude comment about me. That fear has almost always stopped me getting too intimate with just about everyone.

Since my terrible times in my late teens, I have of course had a few relationships which I have let to develop into intimacy, but still I would almost never let any of my partners see me naked, or try to touch me, and for someone to see me erect? Well, that almost never happens; the fear of that is sometimes just too much for me to handle, and have often felt like vomiting with the worry of it.

SUICIDE, A GREAT WAY TO OPT OUT

For a long, long while I went through a really bad time, and thought that one of the only ways of not ever being hurt again, was simply to not be here. To end my life. It made perfect sense. And even today, these thoughts are still very often in my mind; death is one sure way of not being hurt again or not ever going through the emotions of fear, embarrassment and awkwardness of getting intimate and therefore of possibly of being hurt. The other sure way was of course to not get physical with anyone, but everyone wants to be physical! We all want to be desired! I was a good-looking man with a good physique that women desired, and who could easily attract the women that I physically desired. Lovely looking women wanted to get to know me, but the though of me taking my clothes off in front of them often sent me into a spiral of very deep and lasting depression. I did enjoy life though, and I have always tried to experience lots of things like travelling – which has always been an interest of mine – but there was (and still is) a very deep sadness within me; I want to be loved and adored so much, I crav it, but I have tried to keep myself away from it and, in my quiet moments, often thought about (and still think about), escaping this sadness into the void of nothingness, to death.

I have known a few people who have a disability or are disfigured in some way, and who have also had quite intense feelings of depression and of wanting to escape their physicality. I understand them completely; the constant pressure of wanting to being accepted and knowing that you never will is emotionally extremely challenging. And the paradox is that if I become stronger and say to myself; *'I am who I am, and I am beautiful in every way,'* I will open myself up to possibly being humiliated and ridiculed again, which will send me back into the darkness. This is really tough, and especially tough when this humiliation and ridicule comes from something physical and sexual and therefore extremely emotional.

I read on an online penis enlargement forum a father posting: *"How can I make sure my son doesn't suffer from having a small penis, like I have suffered over the years."* He knew what it was like to suffer with a small penis, to be humiliated and to have all the sexual and emotional challenges that are associated with having a small penis, and he was desperate that his son didn't go through the same things.

This is very sad too.

It isn't enough just to be loved; it doesn't change either my cock size, how I feel about it or how I feel about myself because of it. Even if cock size really doesn't matter to someone else, it matters to me and no matter what I have tried I have never managed to overcome these horrible feelings.

SEX ISN'T EASY WITH A TINY COCK

Having a cock slightly less than five inches erect also means that I am quite limited as to the number of sexual positions I am able to perform. For example, a woman sitting on top of me won't feel my cock inside her; I won't fill her up like a larger, longer cock will do and also, because I'm so small I fall out easily. Me on top, in the classic missionary position, isn't a great position for a small cock either because, with body-shapes and legs and hips, not enough of my cock enters her for her to feel it properly, which of course won't happen with a bigger, longer cock. Also, I can't slide in and out easily, as there isn't much of me to slide in and out; if I start to move backwards and forwards, I fall out! So, in this position, if I can, I have to push against the bottom of the bedframe and then what tends to turns a woman on is not my cock inside of her, but my pelvic bone rubbing against her clit. Standing up against the wall is another impossible position for me too, as again, there is just not enough of me to enter her properly, and laying on the side also impossible; I can just about get the tip in, nothing else, and definitely no movement. Her sitting on my lap facing me too is another no-no, as again, when I am sitting, my erection is so small there is nothing for me to go inside her. In fact most positions are almost impossible as there just isn't enough of my cock inside a woman for her to feel it, although from behind, doggy-style, is a bit better, but a lot of women don't like this position and of baring their bum in the air.

And because of the sexual limitations of having a small cock, I do sometimes get quite envious when I see intimate scenes of passionate sex on telly or in the movies; where the girl rips her lover's clothes off and the camera pans down to see her urgently unbuckling his trouser belt. That has never, ever happened to me, even if I have known some stunning women that I would have loved to have had that kind of passionate sex with. The thought of a woman unbuckling my trouser-belt and putting her hands down my pants to grab my four and three quarters inches is just horrific. And watching scenes of a couple doing it frantically against a wall pisses me off too because again, it just can't happen for me. Because of my physicality, I have never, and most likely will never experience these sorts of purely sexual situations. I suppose I have the same thoughts and feelings and emotions about sex as other people who are stopped from doing other things in life because of their own personal physical challenges. The only difference is that my difficulties are sexual and therefore much more emotional. People with sexual challenges are normally much more emotionally affected, because sex and being accepted sexually is so important to the human race. Everyone lives for sex, dreams about sex, fantasizes about sex and wants to have sex! Sex is everywhere and we see people around us in a sexual way; are they attractive and are they therefore sexual? Instinctively humans hunt for sex

– mostly in a good way of course – and it is normal for most people to want to have sex and the feel that someone wants to have sex with them. Sex is the reason you drive across the country to see someone, sex is the reason why you bought those expensive pair of jeans, sex is the reason why women order a salad instead of a burger and fries, sex is the reason why people stay together even though they know they'll never be able to love each other. And when we have a physicality that stops us having sex and doing these very natural and normal things, life becomes very difficult, extremely emotional and quite complex.

SMALLER WOMEN HAVE SMALLER PUSSIES

I remember one time when I was bold enough to get intimate with a tall, very pretty former model. I got chatting to her at a bar and she invited me back to her place for a coffee. We started to get a bit friendly, kissing and cuddling, and then went upstairs to her bedroom. I didn't get naked, although she did, and she then asked if I could play with her first with her sex toy. Not one to refuse such an offer I said of course! And then jokingly said; *"I hope it isn't a big one."* As she lent over the bed to get the toy that was just under the bed, she replied; *"Just normal size,"* and turned to me with this very large dildo in her hand. It was probably about seven inches, thick too, with realistic pink balls. And this was normal size for her; she really said it as though that was the normal sized cock she was used to having. I gulped. Of course I couldn't let her see my little thing after that and, after a little play, made a speedy exit before things went any further. And so, over the years, the few women that I have met and become intimate with have tended to be the smaller, more petite woman than a taller, larger woman, because smaller women naturally have a smaller pussy. There's a lot of evidence that the size of men's cocks around the world compare to the size of women's pussies, for example Indian and Asian women would biologically have smaller pussies to accommodate their men who statistics show have smaller cocks. And the opposite is shown for

African women who have larger pussies to accommodate the larger cocks of their men. And so I know that if I go for smaller, more petite women, they might enjoy my body a little more than perhaps a bigger women would. Like any man, I would love a women to enjoy my body, as I would want to enjoy hers, but a larger, taller, bigger woman would need a much larger cock to satisfy her, and a cock just under five inches just isn't going to do the trick. A tall and very broad-minded woman friend has said this quite openly; five inches is just too small for her, as is six or seven inches. She's a big girl and she needs a big cock to really turn her on. And I am sure, if she is honest enough to say this out loud, there are many other taller, larger women who are perhaps not as open but would probably think the same too. Whereas for a more petite girl, a larger cock might be just too uncomfortable for her naturally much smaller pussy. Also, my small cock looks kind of pathetic and tends to disappear in the larger hands of a larger girl too. With one big hand gripping me, there is very little else poking out the top! Men are, of course, more visual than women and men like to see what's going on, unlike women who are able to get turned on just by touch and imagination, and so the small hands of a petite women around me is so much more arousing to look at than a larger hand around it.

GODS AND THEIR BLOODY HUGE COCKS

The infatuation with penis size isn't a modern phenomenon though, cocks and the size of cocks are well documented throughout the centuries, which is probably why we are still so focused on it today.

For example, in Greek mythology, Priapus was a fertility god, protector of livestock, fruit, plants, gardens and male genitalia (yup, they all go together very well don't they?), and is often portrayed by his oversized, permanent erection, which gave rise to the medical term priapism. Priapism, by the way, is a persistent and often painful erection, not necessarily related to sexual stimulation, that lasts for several hours. Priapism happens when blood that fills the penis during an erection is unable to flow back out of the penis. Great, you may say, but it isn't,! Priapism is actually a medical emergency and if it is not treated within twenty-four hours, your penis may be permanently damaged and you may have difficulties getting it up in the future. Treating priapism isn't a nice thing either, as a needle and syringe is used to drain the blood out of the penis. Ouch! And if that doesn't work, medication may be then injected into the penis which squeezes the blood vessels and helps push the blood out of your penis. Double ouch! And if that doesn't work, wait for it... you will have to have surgery which can involve two things, firstly creating a new route for blood to flow out of the penis or a technique called embolisation may be used which aims to stop the flow of blood into your penis by inserting a small device to block the damaged artery.

Anyway, back to the god Priapus who became a popular figure in Roman erotic art and Latin literature, and is the subject of the often humorous and rather obscene collection of verse called the Priapeia. This big-cocked god was originally worshipped by Greek colonists in Lampsacus in Asia Minor, who revered Priapus more than any other god. Well they would, wouldn't they? The cult of worshipping Priapus spread to mainland Greece and eventually to Italy during the 3rd century BC. Statues of Priapus were often hung over the doorways of houses with warnings threatening sexual assault towards thieves and wrongdoers. The god Priapus' huge cock was used both as a warning and a weapon:

"I am not hewn from fragile elm, nor is my member which stands stiff with a rigid shaft made from just any old wood. It is begotten from everlasting cypress, which fears not the passage of a hundred celestial ages nor the decay of advanced years.
Fear this, evil doer, whoever you are. If your thieving rod harms the smallest shoots of this here vine, like it or not, this cypress rod will sodomize you and plant a fig in you." Marcus Valerius Martialis - Roman poet.

Priapus, the god with the cock, went onto to be

worshipped as a holy icon in much of the world including Egypt, India, Syria, Persia, Greece, Spain, Germany and Scandinavia. In fact, the city of Tyrnavos in Greece still holds an annual phallus festival, which has made the place pretty famous. This is a traditional event on the first days of Lent, where symbols of cocks are paraded through the city. One of the cock devices measuring twenty-five foot (7.6 metres) was actually banned by the organisers of the normally very liberal-minded Edinburgh Festival for being too obscene! There are other well-known annual penis parades around the world, including the Festival of the Steel Phallus held on the first Sunday of every April at the Kanayama Shrine, in Kawasaki, Japan. The penis in the central theme of the event which is reflected in penis illustrations, cock-shaped candy (yup, and then given to children), carved cock-shaped vegetables and decorations. Oh, I have to quickly tell you about the history of this parade... the legend being that a sharp-toothed demon hid inside the vagina of a young woman and castrated two young men on their wedding nights. I do have to question why this woman had two men on her wedding night! But anyway, as a result, the young woman sought help from a blacksmith, who fashioned an iron phallus to break the demon's teeth, which led to the shrine of this iron cock. Another question or two I have is that, well... was this inserted into the woman? Did she agree to it? How big was the phallus and did the iron cock hurt? Nothing like the Japanese veneration of the cock!

Britain's most famous phallus probably belongs to the Cerne Abbas Giant. Dating back to the late 17th century, naked and sporting an erection of thirty-six feet (eleven metres) long, the Giant is one of England's best known hill figures. The Giant and his erect cock is usually associated with fertility and is a major visitor attraction in the region. Yes, renowned for his manhood, people travel from all over to see his massive cock. This is the particular attraction of this particular hill figure, but I wonder if it would be such a big attraction if the Giant had sported a tiny cock? People love looking at big cocks, even if they are carved into the Dorset hillside.

Men and their huge cocks are worshipped around the world and there are also phallic idols found in temples in Mexico, enormous phallus statues found on the Pacific Islands and penis worship was prevalent in India from almost 3000BC, when it was closely associated with magical rites and Shiva. Shiva is worshipped much more commonly in the form of the lingam - or the phallus - and is probably the most widely worshipped male deity in Hindu temples today. Evidence of prehistoric phallic worship can be found in many of the old temples and museums in India and abroad, in the form of stone lingams with several varieties and styles of penis heads, the most famous being the five foot (1.5 metres) high polished black granit Gudimallam lingam in the Parashurameshwar Temple in Andhra Pradesh.

The phallus also played an important role in the cult of Osiris, in Ancient Egypt. Osiris was murdered by his evil brother Typhon, not sure why, maybe just because Typhon was evil? Osiris' body was cut in between fourteen and twenty-four pieces, depending upon which version of the myth you read. These body parts were then scattered all over Egypt. Osiris' other brother Set and his wife Isis retrieved all of them except one, his penis, which was apparently swallowed by a fish, the myth doesn't say whether it was a goldfish or whale. Anyway, Isis (yup, his brother's wife, makes you wonder!) made a wooden replacement of his brother-in-law's erect cock. These wooden erections were then replicated and distributed to several locations, which then became centres of Osiris worship.

In Bhutan the erect penis is commonly depicted in its paintings, and in Indonesia the yoni (vagina) remain common symbols of harmony. In the Sultan's Palace of Kasepuhan, in West Java, there are a large number of lingam / yoni, or penis / vagina carvings along its walls and, according to the Indonesian chronicles of the Babad Tanah Jawi , Prince Puger gained his kingly power from God, by ingesting sperm from the phallus of the already-dead Sultan Amangkurat II of Mataram. What things people do for power!

Talking about power, in accordance with the long-held tradition, the bear on the coat-of-arms of the Swiss municipality of Portein, Switzerland, has a clearly visible red phallus. All heraldic bears in a coat-of-arms had to be painted with bright red penises, or would be mocked as being she-bears and, in 1579, a calendar printed in St. Gallen omitted the penis from the heraldic bear of Appenzell, nearly leading to war between the two cantons. A penis is a symbol of manliness and therefore power.

In the Ecclesia Gnostica Catholica or Gnostic Catholic Church, founded by the obviously eccentric Aleister Crowley, some chapters practice the consumption of semen during the Gnostic Mass. Crowley was an English occultist and ceremonial magician and founded the religion and philosophy of *Thelema*, in which he identified himself as the prophet entrusted with guiding humanity through a series of aeons, characterized by their magical formula. There are said to be several hundred thousand followers of *Thelema* and *Thelemites* believe that humanity will enter a time of self-realization and self-actualization, and I suppose consuming semen every Sunday helps!

The Gnostic Catholic Church is based in America (well, it would be, wouldn't it?), and another North American religion that centres on the worship of the cock is St. Priapus Church, yes, Saint Cock's Church! Founded in the 1980s in Montreal, Quebec, by D. F. Cassidy, its followers are mainly gay men. Like *Thelema*, semen is also treated with reverence and is sacred because of its divine life-giving power and its consumption is an act of worship. Perhaps this is one reason the religion is followed mainly by homosexual men?

And what about the penis in the animal world? There are many species of primates that establish group hierarchy by displaying their erections, and monkeys with a smaller erection cower before the one with the biggest. As many of these species have multiple mates, so the biggest penis is often the one with the most mates. Gorillas however, have one of the smallest penises in primates but mate for life; there is no need for penis comparison or competition from other penises. This basic evolution theory supports the evidence that men with bigger cocks tend to sleep with more women on average than men with small cocks.

Phallology is the scientific study of the penis and the Phallological Museum in Icelandic is probably the only museum in the world that focuses on this science. The museum contains a collection of more than two hundred penises and penile parts belonging to almost all the land and sea mammals that can be found in Iceland. According to its website: *"Visitors to the museum will encounter fifty five specimens [of penis] belonging to sixteen different kinds of whale, one specimen [of penis] taken from a rogue polar bear, thirty-six specimens [of penis] belonging to seven different kinds of seal and walrus, and more than one hundred fifteen specimens [of penis] originating from twenty different kinds of land mammal: all in all, a total of more than two hundred specimens [of penis] belonging to forty six different kinds of mammal, including that of Homo sapiens. Besides there are some twenty-three folklore specimens [of penis] and over forty foreign ones. Altogether the collection contains two hundred and eight-two specimens [of penis] from ninety-three different species of animals. In addition to the biological section of the museum, visitors can view a collection of about three hundred and fifty artistic oddments and practical utensils related to the penis."* In 2011, twelve thousand people visited the museum, which is on average thirty-eight people a day interested in looking at the penises of animals.

Oh, the oldest known species with a penis is a hard-shelled sea creature called Colymbosathon ecplecticos, which is Greek for: 'amazing swimmer with large penis.'

So, society's infatuation with the large penis and it reverence as something to be admired, looked up to and even worshipped is not a modern phenomena, it is steeped in history and biological evolution. But that doesn't help much when you have a small one!

I AM WHO I AM, SMALL COCK AND ALL

As I mentioned earlier, one very nice woman once said to me; *"... it's you I really like, not your cock,"* And I time and time again, as discussed in this little book, I have wonder if these are just the thoughts of a few or is this what most women actually think?

Many times, over the years, I have asked myself if I have been jaded and emotionally traumatised by the women who have belittled me and humiliated me; the nasty women in the world who have just wanted to put me down, whereas I should have listened more to the women that have been nice to me, and who have accepted me for exactly who I am. Am I subconsciously labelling all the women I have met over the years in a negative way just because of the actions of a very few? After all, I am who I am and, despite trying and trying, I can't change the size of my cock; it isn't a muscle that I can build like I can my biceps! So, should I stop trying? Should I stop wishing I was different? Should I stop looking at the ugly side of me and concentrate on the good things? Should I stop looking at the negative sides of my physicality and try to find some positive sides? Should I stop dreaming about doing the things I cannot do sexually, nor will ever be able to do, and just focus on mastering what I can do? Should I stop looking at other men and feeling jealous and envious knowing that they will most likely be much bigger than me, (as almost every man is)? Should I stop seeing this imperfection as something that makes me less of a man - or a person - but try to see how this imperfection actually make me a better person? Rather than being so serious and so emotionally strung-out over my cock, should I try to make light of it and stay chilled? Should I stop comparing myself to others, but just compare myself to the person I was yesterday, and want to be tomorrow?

All of these things are of course easier said than done, but ultimately... should I just accept who I am and simply try to move on? But, is this even possible? Have I carried this burden for just too long, and have I had too many emotionally traumatic experiences, not just by others but from within my own mind, to allow this to happen? Am I permanently damaged emotionally because of who I am physically?

There is a lot of interesting discussions about small cocks on the Internet, with many men embracing their small penis. I even read a story about Nick Gilronan, a 27-year-old UPS Store worker, who recently won Brooklyn's smallest penis contest. Yup, he actually entered a contest for men with small penises... and won! He said: *"The size of a man's penis does not matter for who he is as a person or in a relationship."* He went to say to the website *The Gothamist* about whether small penises have a bad rep: "*Yes. That's the media's fault, I think. For both men and women, the media push out images of people who just aren't, regular normal people. The size of a man's penis does not matter for who he is as a person or in a relationship... Some people let that false sense of body image upset them and they shouldn't be upset at all. Even worse, some people use those false standards and judge other people. It's disconcerting."* And the female reporter he was talking to then blogged and said: *"Hear, hear. The fact is, is that Nick is right - penis size is not the most important thing to a woman."* Tracey Cox, sex expert has long since been an advocate of the fact that size doesn't count said to HuffPost UK Lifestyle: *"If you are worried about penis size, you should know that most women learn very quickly, that if a guy has a big penis he's not going to be much good at sex because he thinks that's enough, and he doesn't need to try."*

There's also a small penis dating website called Kwink, which states: *Little is the new big! Find that special someone that loves your small penis at least as much as you.* Based in La Cygne, Kansas, USA, the first female profile I looked at (limited access, as I wasn't a member... honest!) stated *"I love small cocks."*

And so, after asking myself all of these questions, I must then ask myself; is there a woman for me out there that will like me physically as well as like me emotionally? Or rather, is there a woman out there that will *love my physicality* as much as they will love me as a person? As I mentioned earlier in this little book, I want to one day have brilliant sex with a women that wants to have brilliant sex with me, regardless of how small my penis is. I want a women that will enjoy me being inside her and who will enjoy holding me and sucking me, despite my size and my huge insecurities about my size. I want a woman that will adore me regardless of my physicalities and who will say that they love me and everything about me, unconditionally.

But I know ultimately this will probably never happen... unless I let it happen. I know that I have to accept myself and who I am first, before anyone else can accept me. And I know that I have to love myself and everything about me, before anyone else can.

THE END

Coming soon (no pun intended)...

The Small Penis Society (SPS)
For men 5.5 inches or under

Includes an international dating arena for
women who love men with small cocks!

For further details email:
IvanLittle@RobinBarrattPublishing.com

PROMISCUITY
Compiled and edited by Julie Lovely
ASIN: B00TWKGD3W
£0.99 / FREE Kindle Unlimited

Promiscuity - is a unique interview based project with three women who have led promiscuous lives and the impact it has had on them.

Although in different countries the statistics are slightly different, in the UK and in the US sex-based surveys have shown that most women sleep with between 6 to 8 men before settling down with one long-term partner. A woman is said to be promiscuous if she has slept with over 12 men. But what makes a woman promiscuous and go from partner to partner? Does it stem from their childhood and parental influence; a feeling of being rejected, or physically or emotionally abused? Is it circumstance, meeting the wrong people at the wrong time, and if so why does this continually happen? Is it simply using sex as a form of immediate emotional attachment? Do previously promiscuous women look for specific sexual characteristics or attributes in their partners? What impact does promiscuity have on finding permanent loving relationships? Can previously promiscuous women be honest about their past lives with their partners and if so, what impact does it have on their partners and can they still find long-term happiness?

EROTICA
12 short stories about adult fantasies
By Lily, Terese, Katherine and Julie Lovely
ASIN: B00SDK3ZBU
ISBN: 978-1508643425
Kindle - £1.71 / FREE Kindle Unlimited
Paperback - £4.99

Some wonderfully naughty erotic short stories about sexual fantasies and experiences from the wicked yet enchanting minds of Lily, Terese, Katherine and Julie.

Guaranteed to arouse and awaken sexual expression and a desire to do something just a little bit... naughty!

Robin Barratt Publishing

www.ingramcontent.com/pod-product-compliance
Lightning Source LLC
Chambersburg PA
CBHW070821290526
45795CB00002B/800